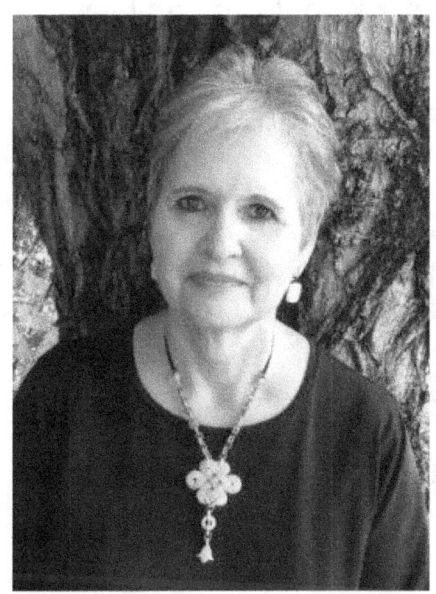

Qigong For Parkinsons: A Conversation with Bianca About Her Complete Healing

Bianca Molle
Robert Rodgers PhD

© *Parkinsons Recovery*

1

Qigong For Parkinsons: A Conversation with Bianca about Her Complete Healing

Contents

© *Parkinsons Recovery*

Qigong For Parkinsons: A Conversation with Bianca about Her Complete Healing

Qigong For Parkinsons: A Conversation with Bianca about Her Complete Healing

Tell us about yourself

BIANCA: I was born in New York and my background is teaching. I spent my last 20 years teaching middle school which was a wonderful, wonderful experience and required tons of energy. On the personal level, I am most proud in my personal life of being a mother and a grandmother. I have two wonderful sons and two wonderful, beautiful grandchildren and a lovely daughter-in-law. I am very pleased that that they are my family. I also have extended family in various parts of the country. Now that I've healed from Parkinson's I have a book, Reboot and Rejoice, and a coaching and consulting website, www.mettamorphix.com.

When did symptoms of Parkinson's first appear?

BIANCA: I was diagnosed in 2008, but probably around 2000 the first symptoms appeared. I had no idea that they were Parkinson's-related because I thought Parkinson's just meant a tremor. The tremor did not appear until about two years before my diagnosis.

I would like to caution readers that that if you have the symptoms I am about to list, it does not mean you have Parkinson's disease. People sometimes want to know all the symptoms and then, upon hearing one, will go: "Oh, constipation, gee I have that. I wonder if

Qigong For Parkinsons: A Conversation with Bianca about Her Complete Healing

I have Parkinson's." Parkinson's is a movement disorder where parts of the body that you don't want to shake and move - like hands, arms or whatever – do move, and parts of the body that would like to see move - like the digestive system and the bowels - aren't moving very well.

The first symptom that I was aware of – although at the time I wasn't aware that it was related to Parkinson's – was world class constipation which lasted for many, many years. Then other things started happening. My handwriting degenerated. Being an English teacher and constantly correcting papers and writing all kinds of editorial comments, I thought that I was just getting lazy and sloppy as I was getting older. I thought I was still in control. I wasn't in control. My handwriting was like chicken scratch because of the Parkinson's. I just kept telling myself that if I just took my time it would look better. That was not the case. It is better now by the way.

In addition to the challenges with my handwriting and constipation, I had aches and pains all over. As the Parkinson's progressed – I didn't know what was causing aches and pains. I could actually feel my muscles being squeezed internally. It felt like they were being pulled and stretched from all directions. It was very painful and very fatiguing.

I had some difficulty swallowing - not so much when I was upright eating as when I was lying down in bed. I would be swallowing in the middle of the night, or not swallowing and choking and waking up to that.

The worst tremor was in my left hand and I am left-handed. I also had tremor activity on the right side. My right leg was the leg that was most affected by Parkinson's. When walking my brain thought I was lifting my right foot but in reality that was not happening as my foot would drag along the ground. This did not happen all the time, just once in a while.

When I would go to "relax" at night in bed my fingertips would curl up toward my wrists. That was something that was difficult. When I was getting a massage one time and the masseuse touched my wrist- my fingertips automatically shot up toward my wrist and curled in.

Another symptom that I think other people may relate to is that there were times when I just had random arm movements. This was prior to my diagnosis because somebody said to me, "Oh that could have been from medication" but I wasn't on medication at the time it first happened. For instance, when sitting in the dentist chair the hygienist leaned over me and all of a sudden, my left arm just shot up and got her under the chin. I was not intending to punch her. I did not know how to explain it and I was so sorry. A month or two later I was diagnosed and wrote a note to her explaining what had happened.

I think because I was trying so hard to keep everything together on a simple physical level I did have some difficulty with cognitive functioning. I have worked with learning disabled students as part of my teaching career and now can really understand what is meant by the fact that learning is terribly difficult when you are trying so hard to keep everything together. I had gone from being somebody who was really a quick-study at a lot of things to somebody who was having a real slow learning curve—if existent at all.

To summarize, the most troublesome symptoms consisted of difficulty with my handwriting, constipation, pain, foot dragging, random arm movements, tremors, finger curling at night, swallowing difficulties and problems with cognitive functioning.

Did you notice a loss of the ability to smell?

BIANCA: Possibly, though it is hard to say. Sometimes people would smell things and I would not smell them but sometimes I would. But then, I get a stuffy nose due to allergies which shuts down my ability to smell. I really do not have a definitive answer.

Qigong For Parkinsons: A Conversation with Bianca about Her Complete Healing

When were you diagnosed?

BIANCA: I was diagnosed April 29th, 2008. At the time it was not a surprise. The tremors had gotten worse and worse. I kept telling myself that I was maybe a Type A, or maybe that second cup of coffee I would drink some mornings was doing it, but when it got to the point where it interfered with eating soup - I really had difficulty getting the spoon up to my mouth without spilling - I made an appointment with the neurologist.

How did your neurologist go about determining you had Parkinson's Disease

BIANCA: There was one very long appointment where he did a number of tests. He explained that there was no definitive diagnosis for Parkinson's. He was 99% sure from how my symptoms presented that I did have Parkinson's. Part of his diagnostic protocol was to prescribe a trial run on the dopamine drug Sinemet. If my symptoms started to abate, then that clinched the diagnosis.

I saw one neurologist several times, then I saw a movement disorder specialist who also confirmed the diagnosis, then I saw another neurologist. My diagnosis was actually confirmed by three different neurology professionals.

© *Parkinsons Recovery*

Did Sinemet offer symptom relief?

BIANCA: Yes, it did. Several months before seeing the neurologist and prior to my diagnosis, I had submitted my retirement papers for teaching. I just knew that I did not have the energy to endure another year in all the pain and everything that I was going through. There were going to be some banquets and awards, and this and that. I asked the neurologist if I could continue on the Sinemet –- which was originally supposed to only be taken for only a two-week trial – until the end of school which was mid-June. I wanted to go out on a high and did not want people knowing what was going on. The last thing I wanted was sympathy. The neurologist gave me permission to continue on the drug till the end of the school year.

I did continue taking the drug for a while longer and then went off it. I was surprised at how much worse I felt when I went off it. I didn't want to return to the dopamine drug because it was very early in my situation with Parkinson's. I wanted to save that for later on because of potential side effects which I wanted to avoid for as long as possible.

When I started having real difficulty without taking the drug, I asked if there were something else I could try. I was given another drug. I experienced such a terrible reaction to taking that drug that I went off it and started taking Sinemet again. I continued to take Sinemet for about another year until I discovered Qigong (chi kung).

It almost seemed like I didn't have Parkinson's as everything seemed pretty good when taking Sinemet during the course of that year. Then little by little I guess I started building up a tolerance or whatever happens. I was at the point when I was going to have to increase my medication if I wanted to have a more full and active life. I really did not want to do that.

What was your reaction to being diagnosed with Parkinson's?

BIANCA: I saw the tremor and so the diagnosis did not surprise me. What did surprise me was everything that came along with the package. I thought the package was just a tremor. I did not realize that it included pain and really being a prisoner in your own body. So, my reaction to the entire package of the Parkinson's syndrome was a little bit of surprise.

It was the first thing on my mind when I would wake up in the morning and it was the last thing on mind when I would go to bed. After three days or so after my diagnosis and after living with these thoughts, I had a conversation with myself in bed one night. It was funny. I had an executive board meeting with body, mind *and spirit. We all got into the room and sat down and listened to each other.*

I said basically, "I'm a teacher. I believe that everything is a learning experience. Parkinson's, teach me. Body, teach me. What am I supposed to learn?" It was about just a little over a year after that that I learned how to heal myself. I feel very grateful for that.

How did you find Qigong?

BIANCA: After being diagnosed I went on a search for information. I bought out all the books on Parkinson's at the Borders Book Store in Marin County, California. I did internet searches to find information about various Parkinson's organizations and support groups. I signed up for a DNA study through www.23andme.com.

Twice I came across quotes about Qigong. One was from Doctor Oz. I don't think he mentioned Parkinson's in particular, but the quote said [I am paraphrasing] "If you want to live to be 100 years old and feel good, do Qigong." There was another reference to Qigong that I found somewhere in the many readings that talked about how all movement was good for Parkinson's, but that Qigong in particular was the best.

I scratched my head because I wasn't even sure how to pronounce it. I thought, "I live in Marin County. If I haven't heard of this, where is it?" It was shortly after that that Qigong showed up in my life. I am very grateful to my friend Jean Adams who convinced me to go to the first "Healer Within" workshop led by Mingtong Gu in Marine County. That was my first introduction to Qigong.

Why did you decide to travel to China to learn more about Qigong?

BIANCA: In answering that question the first thing that I'd like to do is to express my gratitude to the teacher who led me to China, who is Mingtong Gu of the Chi Center here in northern California and to his teacher, Dr. Pang Ming, who is still over there in China.

Mingtong studied under doctor Pang Ming who had set up a medicine-free hospital years ago in the Beijing area. The hospital has since closed down. When I went to my first "Healer Within" workshop on June 19, 2009, Mingtong was planning a retreat in China the following September. I saw a video presentation of where we would be staying. It was such a beautiful, peaceful, serene environment that I decided I really needed to go there.

I want to emphasize very strongly that you do not need to go anywhere. Your access to ultimate good health is inside of you.

The decision to make the trip was in itself in some ways the start of healing because I never did things like that for myself. When I first began thinking about traveling to China I thought to myself: "Only other people do things like that, I don't do things like that." Then I thought to myself: "Why can't I do things like other people? Why can't I step up to the plate and do that? This is my life."

It might be crazy to travel around the world with Parkinson's disease but that is what I did. I was off my medications, thanks to Qigong, at the time that I made to trip. I did not want meds to mask the symptoms that I was working on clearing. I wanted to go on the retreat to China and I wanted to practice Qigong 24/7. I just felt that by doing something that was so out of the ordinary that maybe some other things that were out of the ordinary would start to happen for me too. And, they did!

How long did it take to see sustained relief and then to become symptom-free?

BIANCA: Sustained relief started happening right away. I started feeling one layer of pain strip away the first time that I practiced Qigong at the Healer Within workshop. There were many layers beneath that so it was a gradual process. I knew all along that something was happening.

I started forgetting to take my medication. Prior to Qigong, as the meds began to wear off every few hours, the tremors would *increase. The pain would increase. The tightness and stiffness would increase. When I first started forgetting to take my medications I was concerned. I was still operating on the western medical scale of, "I have to take my medication every so often." Then I realized, "Wait a minute. If my body is forgetting, maybe my body is telling me that I don't need to do that." As I did Qigong and continued to forget to take my medications, I started to feel relief right away.*

The last thing to go was the tremor. The tremor was visible in China and for months after my return, but it became less and less evident. Sometimes tremoring would appear more when I was doing Qigong or when I was at a weekend retreat. This meant that the energy was moving through the blockages – a good outcome to have. The neurologist declared me to be free of any signs of Parkinson's in September of 2010.

Frankly, I think that I'm still healing. Whether I am still healing from Parkinson's or healing from life - I don't know. I just feel better and stronger every day.

Has your first name always been Bianca?

BIANCA: No. The story goes like this. My email for 30 years or more has been Bianca because I was named after my Italian grandmother whose name was Bianca. The name was anglicized to Blanche which is the name many people know me by.

When I got to China, Mingtong and my other four beloved Chinese teachers - Teacher Ma, Teacher Zhao, Teacher Zheng and Linling Xie - could not pronounce "Blanche". I would have accepted being called "Branch" but they could not even come close to pronouncing the name "Branch." Finally I just looked at them and said, "Can you say Bianca?" They all nodded their heads and went, "Bi-anca, Bi-anca." And I said, "Okay, we have a name."

As it turns out, my life changed the same time of my name change from Blanche to Bianca. I went from somebody who was sick and shrinking to somebody who is well and whose life is exploding in all kinds of good ways, much like beautiful fireworks. I like the name Bianca but will answer to either Bianca or Blanche. Just don't call me late to dinner.

What lessons have you learned on the road to your recovery?

BIANCA: The biggest lesson has been to celebrate small victories. So often in our culture we set up long-term goals that we are not going to celebrate until we achieve them. I have learned the lesson of celebrating small victories from being a parent and a teacher. As a parent, I celebrated every little thing my children did. When teaching special education students, I would celebrate every small step forward a child would make.

© Parkinsons Recovery

Do the same thing for yourself. Celebrate whatever progress you make no matter how small or inconsequential it may seem at the time.

I'm working with someone in London, England who has been practicing Qigong for a very brief period time. Her teacher told her that her movements are more fluid. That news is something for her to celebrate. You do not have to start celebrating when the tremors finally disappear. Mingtong, my Qigong master, has said, "A happy cell is a healthy cell." I really believe that.

Maybe it is not that the dopamine produces the happiness, but that happiness produces the dopamine. Think about that. Make yourself happy and you make yourself well.

In line with that I have learned gratitude. I first learned gratitude with the Parkinson's because I knew that my life as I was living it was going to get smaller and smaller according to the prognosis that I believed at the time. As a result, I really appreciated everything that I could yet do. I can do so much more now and as a result, I appreciate all that. I am so grateful that I can pour myself a cup of coffee in the morning and not have to worry about the mug shaking.

I never realized what a piece of work the body really is. It is amazing. Every night before I go to sleep, I try to think of three things that happened during the day that I can grateful for. Most days I find even more. Some days it is a stretch to find two, but most days three come up pretty easily, if not more. I think that being grateful at the end of every day is a wonderful way to make a habit of practicing good health.

I learned to have confidence in my inner-voice and to realize that there is good out there for me. I know I am on the right trail by staying positive.

Learning to love myself has been really important. I thought I was really good at loving other people and I knew I had some work to do with loving myself. I am learning that the more I love myself, the more that I open up to loving others. Bruce Lipton and some other scientists have measured chi energy and have been able to show the benefits of having unobstructed energy running through the body. Love is the best catalyst for making that happen. Love really is the answer.

Why has Qigong produced such amazing results for you?

BIANCA: I would say dedication to the practice. I do not make a secret of the fact that I practice Qigong two to three hours each day and more if I can. It is a dedicated practice, but also a playful practice. I just have fun and use my mind and my body creatively.

Sometimes people get concerned - particularly people with Parkinson's - about doing things the "right" way. They want to visualize everything exactly the right way and then do the movements perfectly. I have to say that I initially didn't do the movements very well. My balance was off. I had trouble following directions. But, my intent was there eight-million percent.

Intent is the most important thing. Set the intention to heal and begin to work diligently at healing yourself. Do not worry about getting it "right." Just keep doing it. Movements will get better and better with practice. I have told some people with Parkinson's – and I'll modify my language – that if somebody had come up to me when I had Parkinson's and said, "You can be rid of this if you jump into an ocean of feces and swim a mile," I would have dived in and said, "Which direction?" It is the intent that is so important. Do not worry about the rest. Everything else will fall into place.

Describe a typical day

BIANCA: I have some healing CDs made by my teacher Mingtong. I keep one in the CD player by my bed. As I go to sleep at night, when I get up to go to the bathroom in the middle of the night and *when I wake up in the morning, I listen to a healing CD. Before I get out of bed in the morning, I will do ten or more minutes of a practice called La Chi which is a simple arm movement and chant which can be done lying down.*

Depending on what the day is (because sometimes I'm called to substitute teach) I like to start the day with a meditation practice and then go into the physical practice. In the past I've started with the physical practice but right now I'm starting with a meditation. I generally complete the different meditation and physical segments in 2-3 hours. Most of the CDs and DVDs run about 40 to 50 minutes long. I fit any Qigong I do on my own (without using a CD or DVD) into my own time slot, but I generally try to practice for half-hour to 40 minutes at a time if I can.

I do shorter segments of Qigong practice if my day is fragmented. The important thing is to just get in the time. I did no less than a combined total of three hours per day during the first two years of recovery. My formal practice time is a bit shorter some days because of all the Qigong related communications I do. Basically, I like to get some practice in morning, afternoon and evening. If I am working in the classroom, I can always get in an afternoon to late afternoon practice. I modify my practice time as the day demands.

Qigong For Parkinsons: A Conversation with Bianca about Her Complete Healing

Has doing Qigong been successful in helping you deal with fears?

BIANCA: Yes. I did not realize that I was constantly holding my body in a tensed position until I started to relax. I did not know that there was any other way. I thought that was how my body was.

Health practitioners say that fear affects the kidneys and that the kidneys in turn have a great deal to do with Parkinson's. Fortunately, Zhineng Qigong presents many ways to work with the organs, especially the kidneys. Little by little, the meditations (particularly the sound healing meditation), the slow movements of the "Lift Chi Up Pour Chi Down" practice and the Standing Meditation have been extremely helpful in calming me down and making me aware of the sensations of my body.

When I first started healing from Parkinson's my hands continued to hook sometimes when I was in bed in the evening. I was getting better and didn't need to do that anymore, but my body memory was still there. I would catch my hands doing that posture. I would have to make a conscious effort to say to my body: "No, just relax the hands. This is not necessary." It was very interesting.

Do you take supplements?

BIANCA: Since I have been healing over the past few years I have done less and less with supplements. For a long time I did take

1200 milligrams of coenzyme Q-10 (CoQ-10) which is quite expensive. That was supposed to be the wonderful thing to do for PD. I understand that Michael J. Fox's group has come out with a study or is publishing the result of a study that says that there is nothing definitive about that. I still take 600 milligrams of coenzyme Q-10 a day just because it is supposed to be good for heart and other things, but I am not doing anything big with supplements right now.

What about your diet?

BIANCA: My diet tends to be healthy. For years I have been eating food that is wheat and gluten-free. I am not fanatic about anything. I'm not going to let anything get in the way of a good celebration. But for the most part, I am careful about processed foods and sugar and that kind of thing. I'm a lot less strict about my diet than I was ten years ago. I watch salt. I use herbs and organic fresh vegetables. But again, I am not fanatic about my diet.

Do you exercise outside of doing Qigong?

BIANCA: Not a whole lot right now. I am a walker and a hiker. Actually, once I healed from the Parkinson's, I realized that some of the pain and problem with my right leg was not Parkinson's-related. Some of it had been Parkinson's related – particularly the dragging of the foot – but I have some other leg issues that I've been working on that are healing beautifully. Part of the healing is that I'm not going out there and hiking the hills like I used to right now. Right now I'm working on healing my leg with Qigong and giving it a little bit of a rest otherwise. I did go out once this week and I will increase little by little.

What other therapies other than Qigong have been useful?

BIANCA: I'm basically what they call a one-trick pony. I investigated many alternatives and couldn't do some because of financial constraints. Some just didn't seem right for me. I still try and get a massage when I can - once a month if I can pamper myself that way. I think movement, any kind of movement, is great. But for me, "Wisdom Healing" Qigong was my salvation. I'm very fortunate that my healing came through Qigong because whatever we need - if we are really looking for it - comes to us. I would have probably had a difficult time managing a whole lot of different therapies so for me, putting all my eggs in the Qigong basket worked beautifully. It still does.

Of the many types of qigong available "Wisdom Healing" (Zhineng or Chi-lel Qigong - all three terms are synonymous) worked for me. I realize other types of Qigong are being used successfully by other people. If someone is interested in exploring my path give it a minimum of three months as the sole practice and monitor the results before trying other styles of Qigong or mixing and matching. Simple is best.

Why exactly does Qigong help?

BIANCA: There is an explanation of Qigong by my teacher at www.chicenter.com. I will paraphrase what I learned from him. The ancient Chinese believed that almost all disease was caused by a blockage of energy. The theory is that illness will disappear by getting energy to move through the body freely. Ninety-six percent (96%) of the energy in the universe is unseen. We see only 4% from our contact with the physical world. Qigong practice invokes this unseen energy. The different movements of Qigong practice and the different meditations of the practice direct the energy to where it needs to go to heal the body. Chi energy also has its own intelligence. Sometimes it naturally goes to places on its own that need to be healed.

Why do energetic blockages form in the body?

BIANCA: I think it probably comes from life patterns. Take for example the familiar "fight or flight" response that becomes a life style pattern. The body tenses up each time. It keeps repeating the same pattern over and over again. Muscles eventually become tense. Blockages in the physical body form. Muscles harden. Qigong is a gradual process which breaks down and dissolves those old, unhealthy patterns. People have been healed from cancer, diabetes, asthma, orthopedic conditions and addictions. It is amazing to look at the diseases Qigong has helped people to heal.

How has your life changed since recovering from Parkinson's?

BIANCA: I have so much more energy now. I just finished a year of volunteering in my granddaughter's kindergarten class and had a great time. I plan to go back next year and volunteer with her first-grade class. As an offshoot to my substitute teaching, I am often called into special education classes where I have started introducing Qigong. Teachers and staff are so pleased with what has been happening in the special education classes that two teachers are interested in having me introduce Qigong to their classes next year. This thing has just taken a life of its own. I am so grateful to have a message to share. I want to bring the message of hope to everyone.

What is on your bucket list?

BIANCA: I don't have a bucket list per se right now. I like watching things unfold and being very spontaneous. I started coaching people overseas. Something that has been on my mind recently is travel overseas to visit the people I have been coaching. So who knows? All kinds of opportunities are presenting themselves.

I am going to be 63 next month. For the first 60 years of my life, fear was the co-author. For the rest of my life, I would like *confidence and joy and a spirit of adventure to be the co-authors. That is what is on my bucket list.*

Do you offer coaching for people with Parkinson's?

BIANCA: Even prior to release of my You Tube video, people were somehow hearing about me. I started getting emails from across the United States. I talk about my recovery and Qigong in the video so I started getting emails worldwide. People from all over the world wanted to know what I did to recover. I started helping and coaching people who had contacted me and requested help.

I make available information about my recovery which is readily accessible. An article about my recovery was posted on the Parkinsons Recovery blog October 19, 2011. Many people regularly practice the first third of my Qigong routine along with me as they watch me doing it on the You Tube video. I post regular blogs about healing and Qigong on my website: www.mettamorphix.com.

What would you want to say to someone who has just been diagnosed with Parkinson's disease?

BIANCA: You have been given a box but you don't need to crawl into it. Jump out of the box and explore. It is possible to reverse symptoms. Work on the fear. Work on the confidence. Work on the joy.

Would you describe yourself as being symptoms free today?

BIANCA: Yes, I would.

What factors played a role in the success of your healing journey?

BIANCA: Everybody will have a different experience as they travel down the road to recovery. For me it was listening to the inner self and not shutting that down. There was a voice inside of me that was coming out very strongly, telling me what would be the right thing to do. I tried to stay positive even after I was diagnosed and before I found Qigong. When people asked how I was feeling, I wasn't going on and on with a long list of everything that was bothering me. I knew no one would want to hear that. To me, it was really important to try to stay socially connected. I did not want to turn people off.

Every once in a while I would get really honest with somebody in the family or someone who was close to me. My step-mother in New York asked me one day how I was doing. I replied, "Well, it's not getting any better. This thing only goes in one direction you know." Right after I heard my own answer to her question I was hit with a lightning bolt. Something inside my head said, "That's wrong. You know that's wrong."

I will never forgot the message that came from a place somewhere deep inside of me - a place that I didn't even know existed - telling me:" You don't have to keep getting worse." I don't know where that thought came from, but I can tell you that listening to my inner-voice was the key for me.

Did you tell friends and colleagues you had Parkinson's Disease?

BIANCA: I chose not to tell my co-workers until after retirement. I did not want the various banquets and award ceremonies to be a downer for anyone. I did confidentially tell my principal about the diagnosis because some of the side effects of the Sinemet drug I was taking included responses like hallucinations.

I wanted to substitute teach after my retirement and knew that my tremor had been noticeable to others. I did not want people getting the wrong impression about the reason for my tremor. After all the dust had settled and the celebrations were over, I called everybody that I thought might be asking me to substitute teach and let them know that I had been diagnosed with Parkinson's. I thought they would be more likely to ask me to substitute teach if they knew the tremor was Parkinson's related rather than alcohol-related.

When I told friends about my diagnosis they probably thought I was an idiot because I said, "Oh, this is a gift. I get to do whatever I want to do now. I can be as lazy as I want. I've worked hard all my life, now I can be lazy." That was how I put it out there.

When friends asked what they could do to help I said, "What you can do to help is to treat me as though I don't have Parkinson's disease." If you're going to go on a hike or do something you think I might be interested in and you are thinking - "Oh no, she has Parkinson's now. She won't want to come along" - call me anyway. Let me make the decision as to whether or not I feel like going that day. I gave them the guidelines so there wasn't a whole lot of difference in how most people treated me. Some people fell by the sidelines a little bit and that was certainly okay.

Did you recover on your own or did you get help along the way?

BIANCA: Help is out there because of the practice. As my teacher Mingtong says, "In a Chi field, one plus one equals three." It is a cumulative effect. I had the motivation and determination to access the chi field of every Qigong practitioner. I now had the key to recovery and unlocked the door on my own. When I got inside this beautiful universe, there was help everywhere.

What would you say to someone who is thinking all this sounds too intimidating?

BIANCA: I came to this whole field of energy work and Qigong a total bonehead. The message that "The universe will take care of you" to me just used to be, "Blah-de-blah-de-blah." It didn't mean anything. Now I know so differently.

Perhaps what I have been talking about sounds a little woo-woo and a little intimidating, but if you are at all intrigued and curious, take a look. I stumbled onto this path and I am so grateful that I did. It is a path well worth exploring.

How to Hear Bianca Molle on Parkinsons Recovery Radio

Visit http://www.blogtalkradio.com/parkinsons-recovery and scroll back to find the show that aired June 15, 2011 featuring Bianca Molle as my guest.

About Bianca

I am a native of Long Island, New York, and remained on the East Coast until age twenty-three. Upon graduation from Hofstra University and a year of teaching high school English, I ventured to the San Francisco area. After several years in Northern California, I moved to LA. I was married and had two small sons when we moved to the Midwest and spent some time in both the Upper Peninsula of Michigan and in Cincinnati, Ohio. I returned to the SF area, Marin County, specifically, in the early 1980's, and have remained in this lovely locale.

© *Parkinsons Recovery*

Qigong For Parkinsons: A Conversation with Bianca about Her Complete Healing

Along with my move to Marin came single parenthood and a full-time teaching career. After acquiring a Masters in Education with a focus on Special Education, I spent a number of years teaching both learning challenged and developmentally delayed students. I may have done that anyway, but received some intense motivation and inspiration from our family situation: My younger son is autistic.

I think that advocating for Justin's autism advanced my learning curve for handling my own management of Parkinson's disease. I was not traumatized by my own diagnosis- it couldn't compare to how I felt as the parent of a beautiful infant diagnosed over thirty years ago with what was then considered a hopeless condition. My relatively smooth sail through Parkinson's I greatly attribute to the "School of Hard Knocks" degree bestowed upon me by life as Justin's mother. (His own progress within the autism spectrum through auditory integration training could be material for another story sometime.) So after receiving my PD diagnosis, I just skipped the shock, sorrow, self-condemnation and self-pity this time, and went straight into self-activism.

Qigong For Parkinsons: A Conversation with Bianca about Her Complete Healing

Much of the self-advocacy was research, where I first learned of Qigong and that it had been reputed to help Parkinson's. In June, 2009, a little over a year since my PD diagnosis, Mingtong Gu of the Chi Center brought Zhineng Qigong to Marin County. Within my first few minutes of my first practice, I began to feel relief. Symptoms gradually abated. In September of 2010 I was declared symptom- of the disease by the neurologist. Over a year later, I just keep feeling better and stronger in all aspects.

I had retired at age 60, in 2008, due to my worsening condition. Now I not only frequently substitute teach; I volunteer at three different schools each week, bringing qigong to two of them. I babysit for my two precious grandchildren presented me by the gifted couple of Aaron and Kathy, my dear son and daughter-in-law.

Most recently, I have begun Qigong wellness coaching with a focus on Parkinson's and other chronic health conditions. I ask people who may entertain the notion of my coaching them to follow a few steps prior to contacting me. Please go to my website, www.mettamorphix.com. There is much useful information there including a link to my book, Reboot and Rejoice, which has been receiving much positive feedback. Then, for consulting or coaching, contact me at: bmolle17@gmail.com

© Parkinsons Recovery

Many blessings to the reader. Haola!

For more consulting and coaching services, and to order Bianca's book, Reboot and Rejoice, go to her website:
http://www.mettamorphix.com